# SIRT FOOD

# RECIPES

*THE ESSENTIAL RECIPES FOR BEGINNERS*

# *Kelsey Scott*

By reading this document, the reader agrees that under no circumstances is the author responsible for any losses, direct or indirect, which are incurred as a result of the use of information contained within this document, including, but not limited to, — errors, omissions, or inaccuracies.

# TABLE OF CONTENT

# INTRODUCTION

Losing weight without always being hungry? This is what the Sirtfood diet promises. What is behind this new nutritional concept - whose success is also linked to the fact that it has become very popular with stars? What does Sirtfood mean? What foods can be consumed with Sirtfood?

## *What does the Sirtfood diet consist of?*

First of all the good news: Sirtfood is also considered a gourmet diet, because both dark chocolate and red wine are allowed - in moderation of course.

The name Sirtfood derives from the protein sirtuin, or "sirt" for short. Sirtuins are a group of proteins that control the important metabolic and cellular aging processes in our body.

Aidan Goggins and Glen Matten are the successful authors of the book "The SIRT Food Diet". Both are certain that "sirtfoods" - foods rich in sirtuins - can reduce pounds, burn fat and prevent uncontrolled hunger attacks. They also help develop muscles. No wonder so many celebrities are passionate about this new food trend - losing weight thanks to Sirtfood.

What are "sirtfoods"?

The goal is to consume as many foods as possible that activate sirtuins in the body. Foods containing tannin are known to stimulate metabolism. The key to success seems to be the high content of polyphenols, tannins, in these foods.

Tannins activate the various sirtuins in the body and thus accelerate the breakdown of fat. These secondary plant substances are found mainly in plant products.

### *The "sirtfoods" foods are:*

apples

avocado

blueberries

broccoli

buckwheat

strawberries

kale .

capers

garlic

rocket salad

sedno

soy

nuts

citrus fruits

spices such as turmeric and chilli

parsley

extra virgin olive oil

red onions

green tea

black coffee

Red wine

dark chocolate

This list can of course be further supplemented.

Very small inconvenience: only 1,500 kilocalories per day are allowed. In the first three days, the ideal would be to limit yourself to 1,000 calories - so that the metabolism is accelerated.

Going into the detail of the Sirt diet scheme, we remind you that it involves two phases. Taken together, they have a total duration of three weeks, after which you can start including meat-based foods in your menus.

Those who want to follow this diet can find numerous ideas in the book The Sirtfood Diet, a volume written by the two experts mentioned above and in which there are several recipes. Sirt Foods are obviously used to prepare them, but also other ingredients, generally easy to find.

Let's talk about the initial phase, which lasts seven days. Among the main guidelines to follow we find caloric reduction, but also the intake of a juice based on cabbage, rocket, green apple, parsley, celery stalks, green apple, matcha green tea (you can easily prepare it at home) .

During the attack phase of this diet, about 3 to 7 kg can be lost. As for energy intake, in the first 3 days it is advisable to keep around 1000 calories per day. From the fourth to the seventh, however, it can be increased up to 1500, taking the juice a couple of times a day.

Phase two, lasting two weeks, does not include particular indications regarding calorie restrictions, but only the fact of consuming a green juice a day and considering three meals rich in Sirt Food. When it comes to these foods, it is undoubtedly necessary to remember that, in principle, they are precious allies for health by virtue of their content of antioxidant and anti-inflammatory plant compounds.

# *<u>RECIPES</u>*

# PRAWN ARRABBIATA

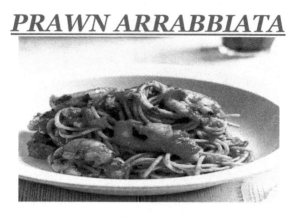

**Prep Time:** 20 mins **Cook Time:** 40 mins **Total Time:** 1 hr

SERVING:2

## *INGREDIENTS*

- 5 oz. Raw or cooked prawns
- 2 oz. Buckwheat pasta
- 1 tbsp Extra virgin olive oil

### For arrabbiata sauce

- 1.5 oz. Red onion, finely slashed
- 1 Garlic clove, finely slashed
- 1oz. Celery, finely slashed
- 1Bird's eye bean stew, finely slashed
- 1tsp Dried blended spices
- 1tsp Extra virgin olive oil
- 2 tbsp White wine (discretionary)
- 14 oz. Tinned slashed tomatoes
- 1tbsp Chopped parsley

# _INSTRUCTIONS_

1. Fry the onion, garlic, celery, and bean stew and dried spices in the oil over medium-low heat for 1–2 minutes. Turn the heat up to medium, add the wine, and cook for 1 moment. Add the tomatoes and leave the sauce to stew over medium-low heat for 20–30 minutes, until it has a decent creamy consistency. On the off chance that you feel the sauce is getting too thick, essentially add a little water.

2. While the sauce is cooking, carry a container of water to the bubble and cook the pasta as indicated by the bundle directions. When cooked, however, you would prefer, channel, throw with the olive oil and keep in the skillet until required.

3. If you are utilizing crude prawns, add them to the sauce and cook for a further 3–4 minutes, until they have turned pink and obscure; add the parsley and serve. On the off chance that you are utilizing cooked prawns, add them with the parsley, carry the sauce to the bubble, and serve.

4. Add the cooked pasta to the sauce, blend thoroughly yet tenderly and serve.

# CHICKEN SALAD

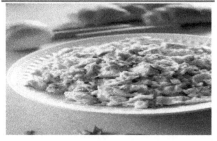

**Prep Time:** 5 mins **Cook Time:** 10 mins **Total Time:** 15 mins

## SERVING:2

## *INGREDIENTS*

- 3 oz Natural yogurt
- Juice of 1/4 of a lemon
- 1 tsp Coriander, cleaved 1 tsp ground turmeric
- 1/2 tsp Mild curry powder
- 4 oz. Cooked chicken breast, cut into scaled-down
- pieces 6 Walnut parts, finely cleaved
- 1Medjool date, finely 1cleaved
- 1oz. Red onion, diced
- 1Bird's eye chilli
- 1oz, Rocket, to serve

## *INSTRUCTIONS*

1. Blend the yogurt, lemon juice, coriander, and flavors in a bowl. Add all the leftover ingredients and serve on a bed of the rocket.

# BROCCOLI AND KALE GREEN SOUP

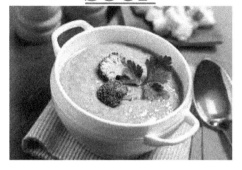

**Prep Time:** 15 mins **Cook Time:** 20 mins **Total Time:** 35 mins

SERVING:2

## INGREDIENTS

- 500ml stock , made by blending 1 tbsp bouillon powder and bubbling water in a container
- 1 tbsp sunflower oil
- 2 garlic cloves , cut
- thumb-sized piece ginger , cut
- ½ tsp ground coriander
- 3cm/1in piece new turmeric root, stripped and ground, or 1/2 tsp ground turmeric
- pinch of pink Himalayan salt
- 7 oz. courgettes , generally cut
- 3 oz. broccoli
- 3.5 oz. kale , cleaved
- 1 lime , zested and squeezed

- small pack parsley ,generally slashed, holding a couple of entire leaves to serve

## *INSTRUCTIONS*

1. Put the oil in a profound container, add the garlic, ginger, coriander, turmeric and salt, fry on a medium warmth for 2 mins, at that point add 3 tbsp water to give a touch more dampness to the flavors.
2. Add the courgettes, ensuring you blend well to cover the cuts in all the flavors, and keep cooking for 3 mins. Add 400ml stock and leave to stew for 3 mins.
3. Add the broccoli, kale and lime juice with the remainder of the stock. Leave to cook again for another 3-4 mins until all the vegetables are delicate.
4. Remove the warmth and add the slashed parsley. Empty everything into a blender and mix on rapid until smooth. It will be a delightful green with pieces of dim spotted through (which is the kale). Topping with lime zing and parsley.

# *SUPERHEALTHY SALMON SERVING OF MIXED GREENS*

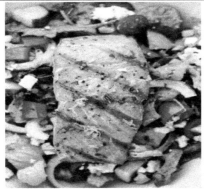

**Prep Time:** 10 mins **Cook Time:** 10 mins **Total Time:** 20 mins

## SERVING:1

## *INGREDIENTS*

- 3.5 oz. Couscous
- 1 tbsp olive oil
- 2 salmon filets
- 7 oz. growing broccoli , generally destroyed, bigger stalks eliminated
- juice 1 lemon
- seeds from a large portion of a pomegranate
- small modest bunch pumpkin seeds
- 2 modest bunches watercress
- olive oil and additional lemon wedges, to serve

# INSTRUCTIONS

1. Warmth water in a level liner. Season the couscous, at that point throw with 1 tsp oil. Pour bubbling water over the couscous so it covers it by 1cm, at that point put in a safe spot.

2. At the point when the water in the liner goes to the bubble, tip the broccoli into the water, at that point lay the salmon in the level above.

3. Cook for 3 mins until the salmon is cooked and the broccoli delicate. Channel the broccoli and run it under virus water to cool.

4. Combine the excess oil and lemon juice. Throw the broccoli, pomegranate seeds and pumpkin seeds through the couscous with the lemon dressing.

5. Finally, generally slash the watercress and throw through the couscous. Present with the salmon, lemon wedges for pressing over and additional olive oil for showering, on the off chance that you like.

# TURKEY ESCALOPE WITH SAGE, TRICK AND PARSLEY AND SPICED CAULIFLOWER COUSCOUS

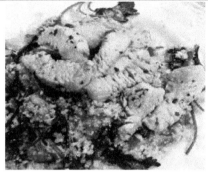

**Prep Time:** 20 mins **Cook Time:** 50 mins **Total Time:** 1hour 10 mins

## SERVING:2

### *INGREDIENTS*

- 5 oz. cauliflower, generally slashed
- 1 clove garlic, finely slashed
- 1,5 oz. red onion, finely hacked
- 1 10,000 foot stew, finely slashed
- 1tsp new ginger, finely hacked
- 2tbsp additional virgin olive oil
- 2tsp ground turmeric
- 1 oz. sun-dried tomatoes, finely cleaved
- 0.35 oz. Parsley
- 5 oz. turkey escalope 1tsp dried sage
- Juice 1/2 lemon
- 1tbsp escapades

# INSTRUCTIONS

1. Place the cauliflower in a food processor and heartbeat in 2-second blasts to finely slash it until it takes after couscous.

2. Put in a safe spot. Fry the garlic, red onion, stew and ginger in 1tsp of the oil until delicate however not shaded. Add the turmeric and cauliflower and cook for 1 moment.

3. Eliminate from the warmth and add the sun-dried tomatoes and a large portion of the parsley.

4. Coat the turkey escalope in the excess oil and sage at that point fry for 5-6 minutes, turning consistently.

5. At the point when cooked, add the lemon juice, remaining parsley, tricks and 1tbsp water to the skillet to make a sauce, at that point serve.

# CRUNCHY POTATO BITES

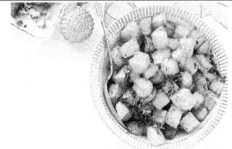

**Prep Time:** 15 mins **Cook Time:** 30 mins **Total Time:** 45 mins

## SERVING:2

### *INGREDIENTS*

- 1 potato, sliced
- 2 bacon slices, already cooked and crumbled
- 1 small 1avocado, pitted and cubed
- 1 tbsp of extra virgin olive oil

### *INSTRUCTIONS*

1. Spread potato slices on a lined baking sheet. Toss around with the extra virgin olive oil.
2. Insert in the oven at 350 degrees F.
3. Bake for 20 minutes.
4. Arrange on a platter, top each slice with avocado and crumbled bacon and serve as a snack.

# GRAPE AND MELON JUICE

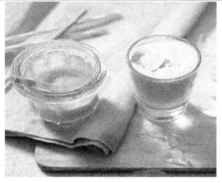

**Prep Time:** 5 mins **Total Time:** 10 mins

SERVING:1

## INGREDIENTS

- ½ cucumber
- 1 oz. youthful spinach leaves stalks eliminated
- 3.5 oz. red seedless grapes
- 3.5 oz. melon, stripped, deseeded, and cut into lumps

## INSTRUCTIONS

1. Blend in a juicer or blender until smooth.

# *CHARGRILLED BEEF*

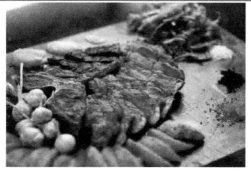

**Prep Time:** 15 mins **Cook Time:** 15 mins **Total Time:** 30 mins

## SERVING:2

## *INGREDIENTS*

- 3.5 oz. potatoes, stripped and cut into 2cm dice
- 1 tbsp additional virgin olive oil
- 0.2 oz. parsley, finely cleaved
- 2 oz. red onion, cut into rings
- 2 oz. kale, cut
- 1 garlic clove, finely cleaved
- 5 oz. x 3.5cm-thick meat filet steak or 2cm-thick sirloin steak
- 40ml red wine
- 150ml meat stock 1 tsp tomato purée
- 1tsp cornflour, broken down in 1 tbsp water

## *INSTRUCTIONS*

1. Heat the stove to 220°C/gas 7.

2. Spot the potatoes in a pot of bubbling water, take back to the bubble and cook for 4–5 minutes, at that point channel. A spot in a simmering tin with 1 teaspoon of the oil and meal in the hot broiler for 35–45 minutes. Turn the potatoes at regular intervals to guarantee, in any event, cooking. When cooked, eliminate from the broiler, sprinkle with the cleaved parsley, and blend well.

3. Fry the onion in 1 teaspoon of the oil over medium heat for 5–7 minutes, until delicate and pleasantly caramelized. Keep warm. Steam the kale for 2–3 minutes at that point channel. 3.Fry the garlic delicately in ½ teaspoon of oil for 1 moment, until delicate however not shaded. Add the kale and fry for a further 1–2 minutes, until soft. Keep warm.

4. Heat an ovenproof griddle over high heat until smoking. Coat the meat in ½ a teaspoon of the oil and fry in the hot dish over medium-high heat as indicated by how you like your meat done. If you want your meat medium, it is smarter to burn the meat and afterward move the skillet to a stove set at 220°C/gas 7 and finish the cooking that route for the endorsed occasions.

5. Eliminate the meat from the skillet and put aside to rest. Add the wine to the hot container to raise any meat buildup. Air pocket to decrease the wine significantly, until sweet and with a concentrated flavor.

6. Add the stock and tomato purée to the steak dish and bring to the bubble; at that point, add the cornflour glue to thicken your sauce, adding it a little at a time until you have your ideal consistency. Mix in any of the juices from the refreshed steak and present with the cooked potatoes, kale, onion rings, and red wine sauce.

# *DATES IN A PARMA HAM BLANKET*

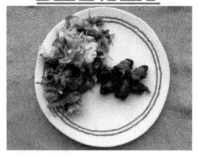

**Prep Time:** 15 mins **Cook Time:** 15 mins **Total Time:** 30 mins

SERVING:12 pieces

## *INGREDIENTS*

- 12 Medjool dates
- 2 slices of Parma ham, cut into strips

## *INSTRUCTIONS*

1. Slice the prosciutto length ways into 2 pieces.
2. Wrap the prosciutto round your dates and keep in place with cocktail sticks.
3. Place the wrapped dates onto a baking tray and bake for around 8-10 minutes.
4. Leave to cool slightly, remove the cocktails sticks and serve!

# VEGETABLE AND NUTS BREAD LOAF

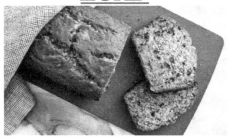

**Prep Time:** 10 mins **Cook Time:** 1 hour 40 mins **Total Time:** 1 hour 50 mins

SERVING:12 pieces

### INGREDIENTS

- 1 loaf
- 175g (6oz) mushrooms, finely chopped
- 100g (3½ oz) haricot beans
- 100g (3½ oz) walnuts, finely chopped
- 100g (3½ oz) peanuts, finely chopped
- 1 carrot, finely chopped
- 3 sticks celery, finely chopped
- 1 bird's-eye chili, finely chopped
- 1 red onion, finely chopped
- 1 egg, beaten
- 2 cloves of garlic, chopped 2 tablespoons olive oil
- 2 teaspoons turmeric powder
- 2 tablespoons soy sauce

- 4 tablespoons fresh parsley, chopped
- 100mls (3½ fl oz) water
- 60mls (2fl oz) red wine

## *INSTRUCTIONS*

1. Heat the oil in a pan and add the garlic, chili, carrot, celery, onion, mushrooms and turmeric.
2. Cook for 5 minutes.
3. Place the haricot beans in a bowl and stir in the nuts, vegetables, soy sauce, egg, parsley, red wine and water.
4. Line a large loaf tin with greaseproof paper.
5. Spoon the mixture into the loaf tin, cover with foil and bake in the oven at 190C/375F for 60-90 minutes.
6. Let it stand for 10 minutes then turn onto a serving plate.

# PANCAKES WITH APPLES AND BLACKCURRANTS

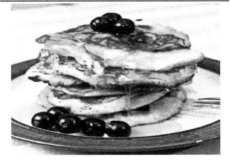

**Prep Time:** 30 mins **Cook Time:** 15 **Total Time:** 45 mins

## SERVINGS:4

### INGREDIENTS

- 2 apples, cut into small chunks
- 2 cups of quick cooking oats
- 1 cup flour of your choice 1 tsp baking powder
- 2 tbsp. raw sugar, coconut sugar, or 2 tbsp. honey that is warm and easy to distribute
- 2 egg whites
- 1 ¼ cups of milk (or soy/rice/coconut)
- 2 tsp extra virgin olive oil
- a dash of salt
  
  **For the berry topping:**
- 1 cup blackcurrants, washed and stalks removed
- 3 tbsp. water (may use less)
- 2 tbsp. sugar (see above for types)

# ***INSTRUCTIONS***

1. Place the ingredients for the topping in a small pot simmer, stirring frequently for about 10 minutes until it cooks down and the juices are released.

2. Take the dry ingredients and mix in a bowl. After, add the apples and the milk a bit at a time until it is a batter. Stiffly whisk the egg whites and then gently mix them into the pancake batter. Set aside in the refrigerator.

3. Pour a one quarter of the oil onto a flat pan or flat griddle, and when hot, pour some of the batter into it in a pancake shape. When the pancakes start to have golden brown edges and form air bubbles, they may be ready to be gently flipped.

4. Test to be sure the bottom can life away from the pan before actually flipping. Repeat for the next three pancakes. Top each pancake with the berries.

# *ORANGE, CARROT & KALE SMOOTHIE*

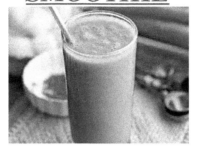

**Prep Time:** 30 mins **Cook Time:** 5 mins **Total Time:** 40 mins

## SERVING:1

## *INGREDIENTS*

- 1 carrot, peeled
- 1 orange, peeled
- 1 stick of celery
- 1 apple, cored
- 50g (2oz) kale
- ½ teaspoon matcha powder

## *INSTRUCTIONS*

1. Place all of the ingredients into a blender and add in enough water to cover them.
2. Process until smooth, serve and enjoy.

# CHOC CHIP GRANOLA

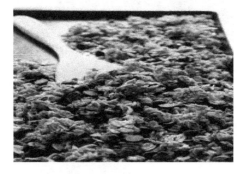

**Prep Time:** 10 mins **Cook Time:** 30 mins **Total Time:** 40 mins

SERVING:15

## INGREDIENTS

- 7 oz. large oats 2 ox. walnuts
- 3 tbsp light olive oil
- 1 oz. spread
- 1 tbsp dull earthy colored sugar
- 2 tbsp rice malt syrup
- dull chocolate chips
- 1 Preheat the stove to 160°C (140°C fan/Gas 3).

## INSTRUCTIONS

1. Line an enormous heating plate with a silicone sheet or preparing material.
2. Mix the oats and walnuts in a huge bowl. In a little non-stick dish, tenderly Heat the olive oil, margarine, earthy colored sugar, and rice malt syrup until the spread has

softened and the sugar and syrup have disintegrated. Try not to permit to bubble. Pour the syrup over the oats and mix all until the oats are completely covered.

3. Distribute the granola over the heating plate, spreading directly into the corners. Leave clusters of combination with dispersing instead of an even spread. Heat in the stove for 20 minutes until just touched brilliant earthy colored at the edges. Eliminate from the broiler and leave to cool on the plate.

4. When cold, separate any more significant irregularities on the plate with your fingers and afterward blend in the chocolate chips. Scoop or empty the granola into a sealed shut tub or container. The granola will save for in any event fourteen days.

# CHOCOLATE CUPCAKES WITH MATCHA ICING

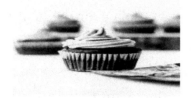

**Prep Time:** 10 mins **Cook Time:** 30 mins **Total Time:** 40 mins

## SERVING:15

### INGREDIENTS

- 5 oz. self-raising flour
- 7 oz. caster sugar
- 2 oz. cocoa
- ½ tsp salt
- ½ tsp fine coffee espresso, decaf whenever liked
- 120ml milk
- ½ tsp vanilla concentrate
- 50ml vegetable oil
- 1 egg
- 120ml bubbling water

**For the icing:**

- 1.5 oz. margarine, at room temperature
- 1.5 oz. icing sugar
- 1 tbsp matcha green tea powder
- ½ tsp vanilla bean glue

- 1.5 oz. delicate cream cheddar

## *INSTRUCTIONS*

1. Preheat the broiler to 180C/160C fan. Line a cupcake tin with paper or silicone cake cases. Place the flour, sugar, cocoa, salt, and coffee powder in an enormous bowl and blend all together.
2. Add the milk, vanilla concentrate, vegetable oil, and egg to the dry Ingredients and utilize an electric blender to beat until all-around joined.
3. Cautiously pour in the bubbling water gradually and beat on a low speed until completely consolidated. Utilize a fast to beat for a further moment to add air to the hitter. The hitter is substantially more fluid than a typical cake blend. Have confidence. It will taste astounding! Spoon the hitter equally between the cake cases.
4. Each cake case ought to be close to ¾ full. Heat in the stove for 15-18 minutes, until the blend bobs back when tapped. Eliminate from the stove and permit to cool before icing. To make the icing, cream the spread and icing sugar together until it's pale and smooth.
5. Add the matcha powder and vanilla and mix once more. At long last, add the cream cheddar and beat until smooth.
6. Line or spread over the cakes.

# TUSCAN BEAN STEW

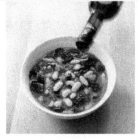

**Prep Time:** 10 mins **Cook Time:** 30 mins **Total Time:** 40 mins

## SERVING:4

## *INGREDIENTS*

- 1 tbsp additional virgin olive oil
- 1.7 oz. red onion, finely cleaved
- 1 oz. carrot, stripped and finely cleaved
- 1 oz. celery, managed and finely cleaved
- 1 garlic clove, finely cleaved
- ½ elevated bean stew, finely hacked (discretionary)
- 1 tsp herbes de Provence
- 200ml vegetable stock
- 1 x 14 oz. tin cleaved Italian tomatoes
- 1 tsp tomato purée
- 7 oz. tinned blended beans
- 1.7 oz. kale, generally cleaved
- 1 tbsp generally cleaved parsley
- 1,5 oz. buckwheat

# *INSTRUCTIONS*

1. Spot the oil in a medium pan over low–medium heat and delicately fry the onion, carrot, celery, garlic, chili, and spices, until the onion is delicate yet not shaded.

2. Add the stock, tomatoes, and tomato purée and bring it to the bubble. Add the beans and stew for 30 minutes.

3. Add the kale and cook for another 5–10 minutes until delicate; add the parsley.

4. In the interim, cook the buckwheat as per the parcel guidelines, channel, and afterward present with the stew.

# TURMERIC TEA

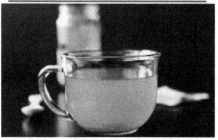

**Prep Time:** 2 mins **Cook Time:** 5 mins **Total Time:** 7 mins

## SERVING:2

### *INGREDIENTS*

- 3 stacked tsp ground turmeric
- 1 tbsp new ground ginger
- 1 little orange , zing pared
- honey or agave and lemon cuts, to serve

### *INSTRUCTIONS*

1. Bubble 500ml water in the pot.
2. Put the turmeric, ginger and orange zing in to a tea kettle or container.
3. Pour over the bubbling water and permit to mix for around 5 mins.
4. Strain through a sifter or tea sifter into two cups, add a cut of lemon and improve with nectar or agave, in the event that you like.

# RED CHICORY, PEAR AND HAZELNUT SERVING OF MIXED GREENS

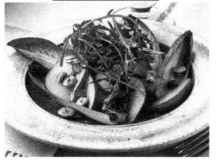

**Prep Time:** 2 mins **Cook Time:** 5 mins **Total Time:** 7 mins

SERVING:2

## INGREDIENTS

- 2 heads of red chicory , or white if not accessible
- 2 ready red Williams pears
- a great modest bunch of rocket leaves
- 1 oz. hazelnuts , toasted and cleaved

**For the dressing:**

- 1 tsp green peppercorns in saline solution, discretionary
- 2 tbsp hazelnut or olive oil
- 2tbsp mellow serving of mixed greens oil, for example, sunflower oil or safflower oil
- 1 tsp sherry or juice vinegar

# *INSTRUCTIONS*

1. Make the dressing. In the case of utilizing green peppercorns, delicately squash them in a bowl with a wooden spoon, or utilize a pestle and mortar.

2. Blend in the oils and vinegar and add salt to taste.

3. Cut back the chicory tail finishes and dispose of any limp or tired external leaves. Cautiously isolated the leaves and organize 5-6 on 4 plates – in the event that they are huge, cut or tear every one into pieces.

4. Eliminate the stalks from the pears and quarter the pears lengthways. Cut out the centers, at that point meagerly cut the natural product.

5. Organize the pear cuts on top of the chicory leaves and spoon over a large portion of the dressing. Pour the leftover dressing over the rocket and season with salt and pepper.

6. Give the leaves a brisk prepare and heap on top of every serving of mixed greens. Sprinkle with the nuts and serve.

# CHICKEN, BROCCOLI AND BEETROOT SERVING OF MIXED GREENS WITH AVOCADO PESTO

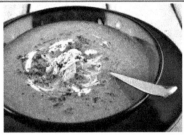

**Prep Time:** 2 mins **Cook Time:** 5 mins **Total Time:** 7 mins

SERVING:2

## INGREDIENTS

- 9 oz. slim stemmed broccoli
- 2 tsp rapeseed oil
- 3 skinless chicken breasts
- 1 red onion , daintily cut
- 3.5 oz. sack watercress
- 2 crude beetroots (about 12.5 oz.), stripped and julienned or ground
- 1 tsp nigella seeds

**For the avocado pesto**

- small pack basil
- 1 avocado
- ½ garlic cloves , squashed
- 1 oz. pecan parts , disintegrated

- 1 tbsp rapeseed oil
- juice and zing
- 1 lemon

## *INSTRUCTIONS*

1. Carry a huge skillet of water to the bubble, add the broccoli and cook for 2 mins.
2. Channel, at that point invigorate under virus water. Warmth a frying pan dish, throw the broccoli in ½ tsp of the rapeseed oil and frying pan for 2-3 mins, turning, until somewhat burned. Put aside to cool.
3. Brush the chicken with the leftover oil and season. Frying pan for 3-4 mins each side or until cooked through.
4. Leave to cool, at that point cut or shred into stout pieces. Next, make the pesto. Pick the leaves from the basil and put aside a modest bunch to top the serving of mixed greens.
5. Put the rest in the little bowl of a food processor. Scoop the substance from the avocado and add to the food processor with the garlic, pecans, oil, 1 tbsp lemon juice, 2-3 tbsp cold water and some flavoring.
6. Barrage until smooth, at that point move to a little serving dish. Pour the excess lemon juice over the cut onions and leave for a couple of mins.

7. Heap the watercress onto a huge platter. Throw through the broccoli and onion, alongside the lemon juice they were absorbed.
8. Top with the beetroot, however don't blend it in, and the chicken.
9. Dissipate over the held basil leaves, the lemon zing and nigella seeds, at that point present with the avocado pesto.

# MORROCAN SPICED EGGS

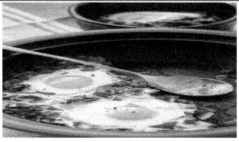

**Prep Time:** 10 mins **Cook Time:** 40 mins **Total Time:** 50 mins

## SERVING:2

### *INGREDIENTS*

- 1 tsp olive oil
- 1 shallot, stripped and finely slashed
- 1 red (ringer) pepper, deseeded and finely hacked
- 1 garlic clove, stripped and finely slashed
- 1 courgette (zucchini), stripped and finely slashed
- 1 tbsp tomato puree (glue)
- ½ tsp mellow stew powder
- ¼ tsp ground cinnamon
- ¼ tsp ground cumin
- ½ tsp salt
- 1 × 14oz can cleaved tomatoes
- 1 x 14oz can chickpeas in water
- little modest bunch of level leaf parsley (0.35 oz. (1/3oz)), cleaved
- 4 medium eggs at room temperature

## *INSTRUCTIONS*

1. Heat the oil in a pan, add the shallot and red (ringer) pepper and fry delicately for 5 minutes. At that point add the garlic and courgette (zucchini) and cook for one more moment or two. Add the tomato puree (glue), flavors and salt and mix through.

2. Add the hacked tomatoes and chickpeas (dousing alcohol and all) and increment the warmth to medium. With the cover off the dish, stew the sauce for 30 minutes – ensure it is delicately rising all through and permit it to decrease in volume by around 33%.

3. Remove from the warmth and mix in the slashed parsley. Preheat the broiler to 200C/180C fan/350F.

4. When you are prepared to cook the eggs, bring the pureed tomatoes up to a delicate stew and move to a little broiler evidence dish.

5. Crack the eggs on the dish and lower them delicately into the stew. Cover with thwart and heat in the stove for 10-15 minutes.

6. Serve the mixture in individual dishes with the eggs drifting on the top.

# CHEESY MUSHROOMS

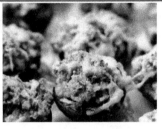

**Prep Time:** 10 mins **Cook Time:** 40 mins **Total Time:** 50 mins

## SERVING:20 Portions

### *INGREDIENTS*

- 20 white mushroom caps
- 1 garlic clove, minced
- 3 tablespoons parsley, chopped
- 2 yellow onions, chopped
- Black pepper to the taste
- ½ cup low-fat parmesan, grated
- ¼ cup low-fat mozzarella, grated
- a drizzle of olive oil
- 2 tablespoons non-fat yogurt

### *INSTRUCTIONS*

1. Heat up a pan with some oil over medium heat, add garlic and onion, stir, cook for 10 minutes and transfer to a bowl.

2. Add black pepper, garlic, parsley, mozzarella, parmesan and yogurt, stir well, stuff the mushroom caps with the mix.
3. Arrange them on a lined baking sheet and bake in the oven at 400 degrees F for 20 minutes.
4. Serve them as an appetizer.

# SALMON AND CAPERS

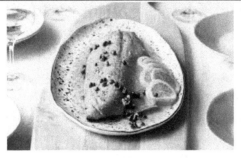

**Prep Time:** 10 mins **Cook Time:** 0 mins **Total Time:** 10 mins

## SERVING:4

## *INGREDIENTS*

- 75g (3oz) Greek yogurt
- 4 salmon fillets, skin removed
- 4 teaspoons Dijon Mustard
- 1 tablespoon capers, chopped
- 2 teaspoons fresh parsley Zest of 1 lemon

## *INSTRUCTIONS*

1. In a bowl, mix together the yogurt, mustard, lemon zest, parsley and capers.
2. Thoroughly coat the salmon in the mixture. Place the salmon under a hot grill (broiler) and cook for 3-4 minutes on each side, or until the fish is cooked.
3. Serve with mashed potatoes and vegetables or a large green leafy salad.

# THAY TOFU CURRY

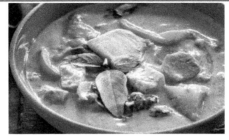

**Prep Time:** 10 mins **Cook Time:** 10 mins **Total Time:** 20 mins

## SERVING:4

### *INGREDIENTS*

- 400g (14oz) tofu, diced
- 200g (7oz) sugar snap peas
- 5cm (2 inch) chunk fresh ginger root, peeled and finely chopped
- 2 red onions, chopped
- 2 cloves of garlic, crushed
- 2 bird's eye chilies
- 2 tablespoons tomato puree
- 1 stalk of lemon grass, inner stalks only
- 1 tablespoon fresh coriander (cilantro), chopped
- 1 teaspoon cumin
- 300mls (½ pint) coconut milk
- 200mls (7fl oz) vegetable stock (broth)
- 1 tablespoon virgin olive oil
- Juice of 1 lime

# INSTRUCTIONS

1. Heat the oil in a frying pan, add the onion and cook for 4 minutes.

2. Add in the chilies, cumin, ginger, and garlic and cook for 2 minutes. Add the tomato puree, lemon grass, sugar-snap peas, lime juice and tofu and cook for 2 minutes.

3. Pour in the stock (broth), coconut milk and coriander (cilantro) and simmer for 5 minutes.

4. Serve with brown rice or buckwheat and a handful of rockets (arugula) leaves on the side.

# MOCHA CHOCOLTE MOUSSE

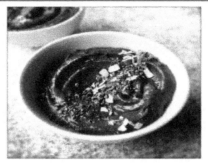

**Prep Time:** 5 mins **Cook Time:** 10 mins **Total Time:** 15 mins

## SERVING:4-6

### INGREDIENTS

- 21.77 oz. dull chocolate (85% cocoa solids)
- 6 medium unfenced eggs, isolated
- 4 tbsp solid dark espresso
- 4 tbsp almond milk
- Chocolate espresso beans, to brighten

### INSTRUCTIONS

1. Melt the chocolate in a huge bowl set over a dish of delicately stewing water.
2. Eliminate the bowl from the warmth and leave the softened chocolate to cool to room temperature.
3. When the dissolved chocolate is at room temperature, speed in the egg yolks each in turn and afterward delicately overlay in the espresso and almond milk.

4. Utilizing a hand-held electric blender, whisk the egg whites until firm pinnacles structure, at that point blend two or three tablespoons into the chocolate combination to extricate it. Tenderly overlap in the rest of, an enormous metal spoon.

5. Move the mousse to singular glasses and smooth the surface. Cover with stick film and chill for at any rate 2 hours, in a perfect world short-term. Brighten with chocolate espresso beans prior to serving.

# TURMERIC PANCAKES WITH LEMON YOGURT SAUCE

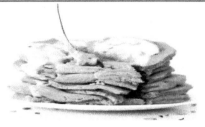

**Prep Time:** 5 mins **Cook Time:** 10 mins **Total Time:** 15 mins

SERVING:8

## *INGREDIENTS*

### For The Yogurt Sauce

- 1 pot Greek yogurt 1 garlic clove, minced
- 1 to 2 tablespoons lemon juice (from 1 lemon), to taste
- ¼ teaspoon ground turmeric 10 new mint leaves, minced
- 2 teaspoons lemon zing (from 1 lemon)

### For The Pancakes

- 2 teaspoons turmeric
- 1½ teaspoons cumin
- 1 teaspoon salt
- 1 teaspoon ground coriander
- ½ teaspoon garlic powder
- ½ teaspoon newly ground dark pepper
- 1 head broccoli, cut into florets

- 3 huge eggs, softly beaten
- 2 tablespoons plain unsweetened almond milk
- cup almond flour
- 4 teaspoons coconut oil

### *INSTRUCTIONS*

1. Make the yogurt sauce. Consolidate the yogurt, garlic, lemon juice, turmeric, mint and zing in a bowl.
2. Put in a safe spot or refrigerate until prepared to serve.
3. Make the hotcakes. In a little bowl, consolidate the turmeric, cumin, salt, coriander, garlic and pepper.
4. Place the broccoli in a food processor, and heartbeat until the florets are separated into little pieces. Move the broccoli to an enormous bowl and add the eggs, almond milk, and almond flour. Mix in the zest blend and join well.
5. Heat 1 teaspoon of the coconut oil in a nonstick dish over medium-low warmth. Empty ¼ cup player into the skillet. Cook the flapjack until little air pockets start to show up on a superficial level and the base is brilliant earthy colored, 2 to 3 minutes.
6. Flip over and cook the flapjack for 2 to 3 minutes more. To keep warm, move the cooked hotcakes to a broiler safe dish and spot in a 200°F stove.
7. Continue making the leftover 3 flapjacks, utilizing the excess oil and hitter.

# *ASPARAGUS*

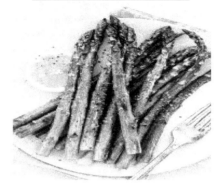

**Prep Time:** 10 mins **Cook Time:** 30 mins **Total Time:** 40 mins

## SERVING:2

## *INGREDIENTS*

- 1 bundle flimsy asparagus lances, managed
- 3 tablespoons olive oil
- 1 ½ tablespoons ground Parmesan cheddar (Optional)
- 1 clove garlic, minced (Optional)
- 1 teaspoon ocean salt
- ½ teaspoon ground dark pepper
- 1 tablespoon lemon juice (Optional)

## *INSTRUCTIONS*

1. Preheat a stove to 425 degrees F (220 degrees C).
2. Spot the asparagus into a blending bowl, and shower with the olive oil.

3. Throw to cover the lances, at that point sprinkle with Parmesan cheddar, garlic, salt, and pepper.
4. Orchestrate the asparagus onto a preparing sheet in a solitary layer.

# BRAISED PUY LENTILS

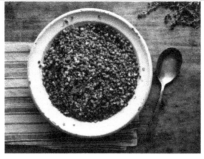

**Prep Time:** 10 mins **Cook Time:** 50 mins **Total Time:** 1 hour

## SERVING:1

## *INGREDIENTS*

- 8 Cherry tomatoes, split
- 2 tsp Extra virgin olive oil
- 1.5 oz. Red onion, daintily cut
- 1 Garlic clove, finely hacked
- 1.5 oz. Celery, meagerly cut
- 1.5 oz. Carrots, stripped and meagerly cut
- 1 tsp Paprika
- 1 tsp Thyme (dry or new)
- 2.5 oz. Puy lentils
- 220 ml Vegetable stock
- 1.7 oz. Kale, generally cleaved
- 1 tbsp Parsley, cleaved
- 0.7 oz. Rocket

# INSTRUCTIONS

1. Warmth your broiler to 120°C/gas ½.

2. Put the tomatoes into a little cooking tin and meal in the stove for 35–45 minutes.

3. Warmth a pot over a low–medium warmth. Add 1 teaspoon of the olive oil with the red onion, garlic, celery and carrot and fry for 1–2 minutes, until relaxed.

4. Mix in the paprika and thyme and cook for a further moment.

5. Wash the lentils in a fine-fit strainer and add them to the skillet alongside the stock. Bring to the bubble, at that point lessen the warmth and stew tenderly for 20 minutes with a top on the skillet.

6. Give the skillet a mix at regular intervals or somewhere in the vicinity, adding a little water if the level drops excessively.

7. Add the kale and cook for a further 10 minutes. At the point when the lentils are cooked, mix in the parsley and simmered tomatoes.

8. Present with the rocket showered with the leftover teaspoon of olive oil.

# KALE AND RE ONION DHAL WITH BUCKWHEAT

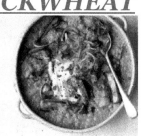

**Prep Time:** 5 mins **Cook Time:** 25 mins **Total Time:** 30 mins

## SERVING:2

### *INGREDIENTS*

- 1 tablespoon olive oil
- 1 little red onion, cut
- 3 garlic cloves, ground or squashed
- 2 cm ginger, ground
- 1 winged creature eye bean stew, deseeded and finely cleaved
- 2 teaspoons turmeric
- 2 teaspoons garam masala
- 5.5 oz. red lentils
- 14 oz. coconut milk
- 200ml water
- 3.5 oz. kale
- 5.5 oz. buckwheat

# INSTRUCTIONS

1. Put the olive oil in a huge, profound pan and add the cut onion. Cook on low heat, with the top on for 5 minutes until mellowed.

2. Add the garlic, ginger, and stew and cook for 1 more moment and then add the turmeric, garam masala, and a sprinkle of water and cook for 1 more moment.

3. Add the red lentils, coconut milk, and 200ml water.

4. Mix everything together altogether and cook for 20 minutes over tenderly Heat with the cover on. Mix sporadically and add somewhat more water if the dhal begins to stick.

5. After 20 minutes, add the kale, mix entirely and supplant the cover, cook for a further 5 minutes (1-2 minutes if you use spinach, all things being equal!)

6. About 15 minutes before the curry is prepared, place the buckwheat in a medium pan and add a lot of bubbling water. Take the water back to the bubble and cook for 10 minutes (or somewhat more if you lean toward your buckwheat milder. Channel the buckwheat in a strainer and present with the dhal.

# *BUCKWHEAT NOODLES - CHICKEN KALE & MISO DRESSING*

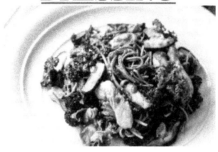

**Prep Time:** 15 mins **Cook Time:** 15 mins **Total Time:** 30 mins

SERVING:2

## *INGREDIENTS*

### For the noodles

- 2-3 small bunches of kale leaves
- 5 oz buckwheat noodles
- 3-4 shiitake mushrooms, cut
- 1 teaspoon coconut oil or ghee
- 1 earthy colored onion, finely diced
- 1 medium unfenced chicken breast, sliced or diced
- 1 long red stew, daintily cut
- 2 huge garlic cloves, finely diced
- 2-3 tablespoons Tamari sauce

### For the miso dressing

- 1½ tablespoon new natural miso
- 1 tablespoon Tamari sauce

- 1 tablespoon extra-virgin olive oil
- 1 tablespoon lemon
- 1 teaspoon sesame oil

## *INSTRUCTIONS*

1. Carry a medium pot of water to bubble. Add the kale and cook for 1 moment, until somewhat withered. Eliminate and put in a safe spot, yet save the water and take it back to the bubble. Add the soba noodles and cook as indicated by the bundle. Flush under virus water and put it in a safe spot.

2. Meanwhile, sear the shiitake mushrooms in a little ghee or coconut oil (about a teaspoon) for 2-3 minutes, until delicately sautéed on each side. Sprinkle with ocean salt and put in a safe spot.

3. In a similar griddle, heat more coconut oil or ghee over medium-high heat. Sauté onion and stew for 2-3 minutes, and afterward, add the chicken pieces.

4. Cook 5 minutes over medium heat, mixing multiple times. At that point, add the garlic, tamari sauce, and a little sprinkle of water. Cook for a further 2-3 minutes, mixing as often as possible until chicken is cooked through.

5. At last, add the kale and soba noodles and throw through the chicken to heat up.

6. Mix the miso dressing and shower over the noodles directly toward the finish of cooking. This way, you will keep every one of those valuable probiotics in the miso alive and dynamic.

# VIETNAMESE TURMERIC FISH WITH HERBS AND MANGO SAUCE

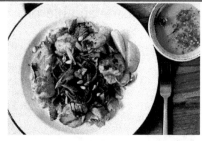

**Prep Time:** 15 mins **Cook Time:** 30 mins **Total Time:** 45 mins

SERVING:4

## *INGREDIENTS*

### Fish
- ¼ lbs new cod fish, boneless and skinless, cut into
- 2-inch piece wide that are about ½ inch thick
- 2 tbsp coconut oil to sear the fish (in addition to a couple of more tablespoon if important)
- Small spot of ocean salt to taste

  **Fish marinade:** (Marinate for at any rate 1 hr. or then again as long as for the time being)
- 1 tbsp turmeric powder
- 1 tsp ocean salt
- 1 tbsp Chinese cooking wine (Alt. dry sherry)
- 2 tsp minced ginger
- 2 tbsp olive oil

### Implanted Scallion and Dill Oil:

- 2 cups scallions (cut into long slender shape)
- 2 cups of new dill
- Pinch of ocean salt to taste.

### Mango plunging sauce:

- 1 medium estimated ready mango
- 2 tbsp rice vinegar
- Juice of ½ lime
- 1 garlic clove
- 1 tsp dry red stew pepper (mix in prior to serving)

### More Ingredients:

- Fresh cilantro (as much as you prefer)
- Lime juice (as much as you can imagine)
- Nuts (cashew or pine nuts)

### *INSTRUCTIONS*

1. Marinate the fish for at any rate 1 hr. or then again as long as for the time being.
2. Spot all Ingredients under "Mango Dipping Sauce" into a food processor and mix until wanted consistency.

### To Pan-Fry The Fish:

1. Heat 2 tbsp of coconut oil in a non-stick enormous griddle over high warmth. At the point when hot, add the pre-marinated fish. Note: place the fish cuts into the skillet independently and separate to at least two groups to sauté if important.

2. You ought to hear a noisy sizzle, after which you can diminish the warmth to medium-high.

3. Try not to turn or move the fish until you see a brilliant earthy colored tone as an afterthought, around 5 minutes. Season with a touch of ocean salt. Add more coconut oil to sear the fish if vital.

4. When the fish is in brilliant earthy colored tone cautiously turn the fish to broil on the opposite side. Whenever it's done, move to an enormous plate. Note: There should be some oil left in the skillet. We utilize the rest of the oil to make scallion and dill implanted oil.

**To Make The Scallion And Dill Infused Oil**:

1. Utilize the rest of the oil in the skillet over medium-high warmth, add 2 cups of scallions and 2 cups of dill. Mood killer the warmth whenever you have added the scallions and dill. Give them a delicate throw just until the scallions and dill have withered, around 15 seconds. Season with a scramble of ocean salt.

2. Pour the scallion, dill, and implanted oil over the fish and present with mango plunging sauce with new cilantro, lime, and nuts.

# SIRT CHILI AND MEAT

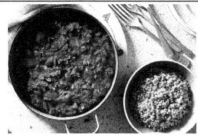

**Prep Time:** 20 mins **Cook Time:** 1hour **Total Time:** 1 hour 40mins

## SERVING:4

## *INGREDIENTS*

- 1 red onion, finely hacked
- 3 garlic cloves, finely hacked
- 2 10,000 foot chillies, finely hacked
- 1 tbsp additional virgin olive oil
- 1 tbsp ground cumin
- 1 tbsp ground turmeric
- 14 oz. lean minced hamburger (5 percent fat)
- 150ml red wine
- 1 red pepper, cored, seeds eliminated and cut into scaled down pieces
- 2x 14 oz. tins cleaved tomatoes
- 1 tbsp tomato purée
- 1 tbsp cocoa powder
- 5 oz. tinned kidney beans
- 300ml meat stock

- 0.2 oz. coriander, cleaved
- 0.2 oz. parsley, cleaved
- 11.5 oz. buckwheat

### *INSTRUCTIONS*

1. In a meal, fry the onion, garlic and stew in the oil over a medium warmth for 2-3 minutes, at that point add the flavors and cook for a moment.

2. Add the minced meat and earthy colored over a high warmth. Add the red wine and permit it to rise to lessen it considerably.

3. Add the red pepper, tomatoes, tomato purée, cocoa, kidney beans and stock and leave to stew for 60 minutes.

4. You may need to add a little water to accomplish a thick, tacky consistency. Not long prior to serving, mix in the hacked spices.

5. In the interim, cook the buckwheat as indicated by the parcel guidelines and present with the stew.

# *SPROUTS AND APPLES SNACK SALAD*

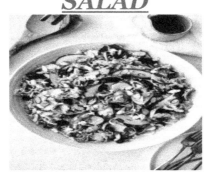

**Prep Time:** 10 mins **Cook Time:** 10 mins **Total Time:** 20 mins

SERVING:6

## *INGREDIENTS*

- 1-pound Brussels sprouts, shredded
- 1 cup walnuts, chopped
- 1 apple, cored and cubed
- 1 red onion, chopped

**For the salad dressing:**
- 3 tablespoons red vinegar
- 1 tablespoon mustard
- ½ cup olive oil
- 1 garlic clove, minced
- black pepper to the taste

## *INSTRUCTIONS*

1. In a salad bowl, mix sprouts with apple, onion and walnuts.
2. In another bowl, mix vinegar with mustard, oil, garlic, and pepper and whisk really well.
3. Add the dressing to your salad, toss well and serve as a snack.

# COCONUT CURRY

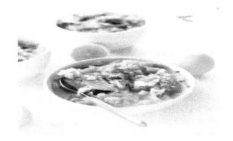

**Prep Time:** 10 mins **Cook Time:** 20 mins **Total Time:** 30 mins

## SERVING:4

### INGREDIENTS

- 400g (14oz) tinned chopped tomatoes
- 25g (1oz) fresh coriander (cilantro) chopped
- 3 red onions, finely chopped
- 3 cloves of garlic, crushed
- 2 bird's eye chilies
- ½ teaspoon ground coriander (cilantro)
- ½ teaspoon turmeric
- 400mls (14fl oz) coconut milk
- 1 tablespoons olive oil
- Juice of 1 lime

### INSTRUCTIONS

1. Place the onions, garlic, tomatoes, chilies, lime juice, turmeric, ground coriander (cilantro), chilies and half

of the fresh coriander (cilantro) into a blender and blitz until you have a smooth curry paste.

2. Heat the olive oil in a frying pan, add the paste and cook for 2 minutes.

3. Stir in the coconut milk and warm it thoroughly. Stir in the fresh coriander (cilantro).

4. Serve with rice

# COURGETTE SPAGHETTI WITH SHRIMPS

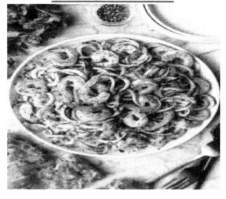

**Prep Time:** 10 mins **Cook Time:** 20 mins **Total Time:** 30 mins

SERVING:2

## INGREDIENTS

- 21.77 oz. of Shrimp
- 2 courgettes
- 1 lemon juice
- 1 stew
- Olive oil q.s.
- 4 cloves of garlic Coriander q.s.
- White pepper q.s.
- White wine q.s.
- Refined salt q.s.
- Coarse salt q.s

# INSTRUCTIONS

1. Start by washing the courgette and cutting into slight, long strips (utilize a winding vegetable chopper).

2. In a bowl place the courgette, season with salt and pepper. Save.

3. Peel the shrimp and sauté in a griddle with olive oil, stew and garlic. Season with coarse salt, pepper and revive with some white wine.

4. After the shrimps are cooked, add the lemon juice and the slashed coriander.

5. Add the courgette and let it cook for a couple of moments.

6. Remove and serve right away.

# MEDJOOL NUTS AND DATES GRANOLA

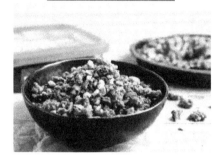

**Prep Time:** 5 mins **Cook Time:** 5 mins **Total Time:** 10 mins

SERVING:1

## INGREDIENTS

- 1 cup of oat chips
- 3 tbsp of nectar
- 6 pecans
- 2 tablespoons of dates

## INSTRUCTIONS

1. In a plate, blend the oats, nuts and nectar.
2. Bake in a preheated stove at 180°C until toasted and fresh.
3. Remove the blend from the broiler and add the dates.

# TURKEY STEAK WITH SPICY CAULIFLOWER COUSCOUS

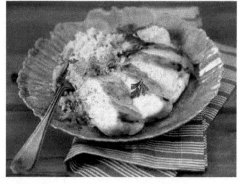

**Prep Time:** 20 mins **Cook Time:** 50 mins **Total Time:** 1 hour 10 mins

## SERVING:2

### INGREDIENTS

- 4-6 turkey steaks
- 1 cauliflower
- 1 red onion
- 2 chillies
- 2 tbsp of ground turmeric
- 1 foot of parsley
- 1 lemon juice
- 2 garlic cloves
- Olive oil q.s.
- salt and pepper q.s.

# *INSTRUCTIONS*

1. Season the turkey steaks with somewhat salt, pepper and lemon juice.

2. To make the couscous, place a crude bloom in a mincer, cutting it daintily until it would appear that couscous.

3. Sauté the garlic, red onion and stew with a touch of olive oil until it picks up shading. Add the saffron and the cauliflower and cook for 1 moment. Eliminate and add the parsley.

   - Grill the turkey steaks.
   - Serve them joined by the couscous

4. **<u>Green tea + lemon:</u>** Green tea consumers can expect various medical advantages given that devouring this valued drink is connected with less malignant growth, coronary illness, diabetes and osteoporosis. These medical advantages can be clarified by its extraordinary substance of plant intensifies called catechins, and particularly a sort called epigallocatechin gallate (EGCG). Adding a crush of lemon juice to your green tea, which is plentiful in nutrient C, serves to essentially build the measure of catechins that get consumed into the body.

5. **<u>Pureed tomatoes + additional virgin olive oil:</u>** Lycopene is the carotenoid answerable for the dark red shade of tomatoes, and its utilization is connected with a diminished danger of specific malignancies (most

outstandingly malignancy of the prostate), cardiovascular illness, osteoporosis, and in any event, shielding the skin from the harming impacts of the sun. The main thing to think about lycopene is that cooking and handling tomatoes drastically builds the measure of lycopene that the body can retain. The second is that the presence of fat further expands lycopene retention. So collaborating your tomato-based dishes with a liberal sprinkle of additional virgin olive oil bodes well.

6. **Turmeric + dark pepper:** Turmeric, the brilliant yellow zest ever-present in customary Indian cooking, is the subject of extreme logical investigation for its enemy of malignancy properties, it's capability to lessen aggravation in the body, and in any event, for fighting off dementia. This is accepted to be essentially because of its dynamic constituent curcumin. In any case, the issue with curcumin is that it is ineffectively consumed by the body. In any case, adding dark pepper expands its assimilation, making them the ideal zest twofold act. Cooking turmeric in fluid, and adding fat, further assists with curcumin assimilation.

7. **Broccoli + mustard:** its an obvious fact that broccoli is beneficial for us, with benefits including diminishing disease hazard. Broccoli's principle malignancy preventive fixing is sulforaphane. This is shaped when we eat broccoli by the activity of a catalyst found in

broccoli called myrosinase. In any case, cooking broccoli – particularly over-cooking it – starts to annihilate the myrosinase chemical, lessening the measure of sulforaphane that can be made. Truth be told, in case we're not cautious, we can cook the advantages directly out of broccoli. In any case, for the individuals who like their broccoli very much cooked (as opposed to gently steamed for 2 to 4 minutes), including other regular wellsprings of myrosinase, for example, from mustard or horseradish, implies that sulforaphane can in any case be made.

8. **Serving of mixed greens + avocado**: Green verdant vegetables, for example, kale, spinach and watercress, are pressed brimming with wellbeing advancing carotenoids, for example, resistant fortifying beta-carotene and eye-accommodating lutein. Nonetheless, when eaten crude, as servings of mixed greens, these carotenoids are more hard to ingest. Yet, the option of some fat can truly assist with that and adding avocado, wealthy in monounsaturated fat, to a plate of mixed greens, has been appeared to drastically expand the quantity of carotenoids that can be ingested.

# MATCHA WITH VANILLA

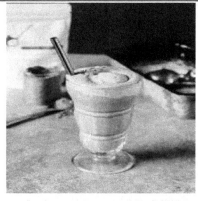

**Prep Time:** 5 mins **Cook Time:** 5 mins **Total Time:** 10 mins

SERVING:1

## INGREDIENTS

- ½ tsp matcha powder
- seeds from a large portion of a vanilla unit

## INSTRUCTIONS

1. Heat up the pot at that point empty 100ml of the water into an estimating container.
2. Empty a large portion of the high temp water into a little bowl, to warm it, at that point add the matcha powder and vanilla seeds to the remainder of the water in the container.

3. Whisk the blend with a bamboo coordinate whisk or smaller than normal electric speed until it's smooth, protuberance free and marginally bubbly.
4. Dispose of the water in the warmed tea bowl, at that point pour in the readied matcha tea.

# *KALE WITH LEMON TAHINI DRESSING*

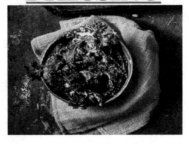

**Prep Time:** 5 mins **Cook Time:**5 mins **Total Time:** 10 mins

SERVING:1

## *INGREDIENTS*

- juice 1 lemon (around 3 tbsp juice)
- 1 garlic clove , squashed
- 1.7 oz. tahini
- 1 tbsp olive oil 7 oz. kale

## *INSTRUCTIONS*

1. To start with, make the dressing. Put the lemon juice, garlic, tahini and 50ml virus water in a little bowl.
2. Blend well to frame a free dressing and season to taste. (Try not to stress on the off chance that it isolates from the outset – as you mix it will meet up.)

3. Warm the oil in an enormous griddle and sautéed food the kale for 3 mins. Add a large portion of the dressing to the skillet and cook for a further 30 secs.

4. Move to a serving bowl and shower over the leftover dressing.

# MALABAR PRAWNS

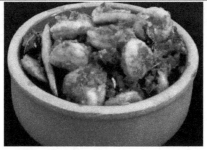

**Prep Time:** 5 mins **Cook Time:**5 mins **Total Time:** 10 mins

## SERVING:1

### *INGREDIENTS*

- 14 oz. crude ruler prawns
- 2 tsp turmeric
- 3-4 tsp Kashmiri bean stew powder
- 4 tsp lemon juice , in addition to a crush
- 1.5oz. ginger , half stripped and ground, half finely cut into   matchsticks
- 1 tbsp vegetable oil
- 4 curry leaves
- 2-4    green chillies , split and deseeded
- 1 onion , finely cut
- 1 tsp broke dark pepper
- 1.5 oz. new coconut , ground
- ½ little bundle coriander , leaves as it were

# INSTRUCTIONS

2. Flush the prawns in virus water and wipe off. Throw them with the turmeric, stew powder, lemon squeeze and ground ginger and put in a safe spot.

3. Warmth the oil in a container and add the curry leaves, stew, cut ginger and onion. Cook until clear, around 10 mins, at that point add the dark pepper.

4. Throw the prawns in with any marinade, and sautéed food until prepared, around 2 mins. Season whenever required and add a crush of lemon juice.

5. Serve sprinkled with the coconut and coriander leaves.

# DILL AND BELL PEPPERS SNACK

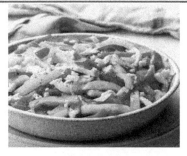

**Prep Time:** 10 mins **Cook Time:** 15 mins **Total Time:** 25 mins

SERVING:4

## INGREDIENTS

- 2 tablespoons dill, chopped
- 1 yellow onion, chopped
- 1 pound multi colored bell peppers, cut into halves, seeded and cut into thin strips
- 3 tablespoons extra virgin olive oil
- 2 and ½ tablespoons white vinegar
- Black pepper to the taste

## INSTRUCTIONS

1. In a salad bowl, mix bell peppers with onion, dill, pepper, oil, and vinegar and toss to coat.
2. Divide into small bowls and serve as a snack.

# SPICY PUMPKIN SEEDS BOWL

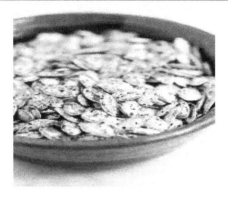

**Prep Time:** 0 mins **Cook Time:** 30 mins **Total Time:** 30 mins

SERVING:6

## *INGREDIENTS*

- ½ tablespoon chili powder
- ½ teaspoon cayenne pepper
- 2 cups pumpkin seeds
- 2 teaspoons lime juice

## *INSTRUCTIONS*

1. Spread pumpkin seeds on a lined baking sheet, add lime juice, cayenne and chili powder, and toss well.
2. Put it in the oven and roast at 275 degrees F for 20 minutes. Divide into small bowls and serve as a snack.

# *SUMMER BERRY SMOOTHIE*

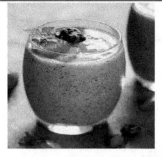

**Prep Time:** 20 mins **Cook Time:** 0 mins **Total Time:** 20 mins

## SERVING:6

## *INGREDIENTS*

- 50g (2oz) blueberries
- 50g (2oz) strawberries
- 25g (1oz) blackcurrants
- 25g (1oz) red grapes
- 1 carrot, peeled
- 1 orange, peeled
- Juice of 1 lime

## *INSTRUCTIONS*

1. Place all of the ingredients into a blender and cover them with water.
2. Blitz until smooth.

# AMAZING GARLIC AIOLI

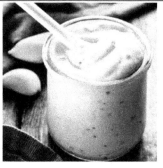

**Prep Time:** 10 mins **Cook Time:** 0 mins **Total Time:** 10 mins

## SERVING:4

## *INGREDIENTS*

- ½ cup mayonnaise, low fat and low sodium
- 2 garlic cloves, minced
- Juice of 1 lemon
- 1 tablespoon fresh-flat leaf Italian parsley, chopped
- 1 teaspoon chives, chopped
- Salt and pepper to taste

## *INSTRUCTIONS*

1. Add mayonnaise, garlic, parsley, lemon juice, chives and season with salt and pepper.
2. Blend until combined well.
3. Pour into refrigerator and chill for 30 minutes. Serve and use as needed!

# TURKEY AND VEGETABLES STROGANOFF

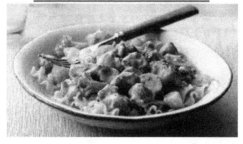

**Prep Time:** 10 mins **Cook Time:** 30 mins **Total Time:** 40 mins

SERVING:2

## INGREDIENTS

- 2 turkey steaks cut into strips
- 1 little red onion cut into half moons
- 1 container of cut mushrooms
- 1/2 cut cabbage
- 1 cut cucumber
- 100ml of light coconut drink
- 2 tablespoons of tomato glue
- 2 tsp of olive oil
- Salt q.s. Pepper q.s.

## INSTRUCTIONS

1. Season the turkey with salt and pepper.
2. Sauté the onion.

3. Add the vegetables, season with salt and cook for around 10 minutes or until everything is cooked.
4. Remove the vegetables from the dish and save.
5. Place the turkey in the skillet and let it cook well on the two sides. Add the vegetables in the skillet once more.
6. Add the coconut milk and tomato glue. Allow it to cook on low warmth for a
7. couple of moments.
8. Taste and, if fundamental, correct the flavors. Remove and serve right away.

# TURMERIC SWEET POTATO WEDGES

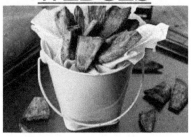

**Prep Time:** 15 mins **Cook Time:** 25 mins **Total Time:** 40 mins

SERVING:2

## INGREDIENTS

- 1 big yam, washed well and dried
- 2 tbspn additional virgin olive oil
- 1 tsp ground turmeric
- 1/2 tsp ground cinnamon (discretionary)
- 1/2 tsp earthy colored sugar
- 1/2 tsp fine ocean salt
- Newly ground pepper

## INSTRUCTIONS

1. Preheat stove to 200 degrees.
2. Line an enormous heating sheet with foil or material paper (best not to utilize a silicone preparing sheet as the turmeric will stain it – and your hands – yellow).
3. Cut potato into wedges or strips. Spot into a huge bowl.

4. Blend the oil and any remaining fixings in a huge bowl at that point, utilizing a huge spoon or utensils, add the potato wedges and throw until equally covered.

5. Spot potato wedges onto preparing sheet.

6. Prepare for roughly 20 minutes, flip, and heat an extra 10 – 20 minutes until fresh.

# CHICKEN, SPINACH AND FLAX MUFFINS

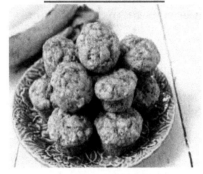

**Prep Time:** 20 mins **Cook Time:** 40 mins **Total Time:** 1 hour

SERVING:4

## INGREDIENTS

- 4 eggs
- 1 red onion
- 2 cups of spinach
- 2 ground carrots
- 1/2 little diced barbecued chicken breast
- 2 tablespoons of flax seeds
- Salt q.s.
- 1 tbsp of cleaved chives
- Extra virgin olive oil q.s.

# *INSTRUCTIONS*

1. Preheat the stove to 170° and oil the biscuit molds with a little olive oil. In a skillet, sauté an onion with a little olive oil.
2. Add a ground carrot and cook for around 5 minutes.
3. Meanwhile, in a bowl, beat the eggs with a spot of salt.
4. Add the chicken and the vegetables to the eggs and mix well. Place the chives and the flax seeds and mix.
5. Place the combination in the molds and heat for around 20 minutes or until cooked.

# *MUNG BEANS SNACK SALAD*

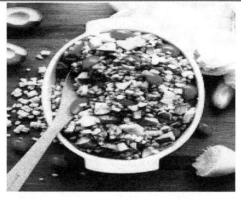

**Prep Time:** 10 mins **Cook Time:** 10 mins **Total Time:** 20 mins

SERVING:6

## *INGREDIENTS*

- 2 cups tomatoes, chopped
- 2 cups cucumber, chopped
- 3 cups mixed greens
- 2 cups mung beans, sprouted
- 2 cups clover sprouts

### For the salad dressing:
- 1 tablespoon cumin, ground
- 1 cup dill, chopped
- 4 tablespoons lemon juice
- 1 avocado, pitted, peeled and roughly chopped
- 1 cucumber, roughly chopped

## *INSTRUCTIONS*

1. In a salad bowl, mix tomatoes with 2 cups cucumber, greens, clover and mung sprouts.

2. In your blender, mix cumin with dill, lemon juice, 1 cucumber, and avocado and blend really well

3. Add the blended cream to your salad, toss well, and serve as a snack.

# ZUCCHINI BOWLS

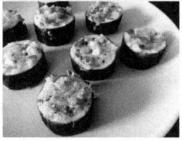

**Prep Time:** 10 mins **Cook Time:** 30 mins **Total Time:** 40 mins

SERVING:12

## INGREDIENTS

- Cooking spray
- ½ cup dill, chopped
- 1 egg
- ½ cup whole wheat flour
- Black pepper to the taste
- 1 yellow onion, chopped
- 2 garlic cloves, minced
- 3 zucchinis, grated

## INSTRUCTIONS

1. In a bowl, mix zucchinis with garlic, onion, flour, pepper, egg, and dill and stir well.
2. Shape the mix into 12 portions with the help of small bowls and arrange them on a lined baking sheet.

3. Grease them with some cooking spray and bake at 400 degrees F for 20 minutes, flipping them halfway.
4. Serve at room temperature as snacks.

# GREEN OMELET

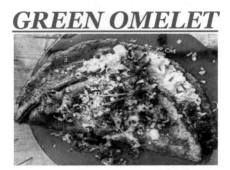

**Prep Time:** 10 mins **Cook Time:** 5 mins **Total Time:** 15 mins

SERVING:12

## *INGREDIENTS*

- 2 large eggs, at room temperature
- 1 shallot, peeled and chopped
- Handful arugula
- 3 sprigs of parsley, chopped
- 1 tsp extra virgin olive oil
- Salt and black pepper

## *INSTRUCTIONS*

1. Beat the eggs in a small bowl and set aside. Sauté the shallot for 5 minutes with a bit of the oil, on low-medium heat. Pour the eggs in the pans, stirring the mixture for just a second.

2. The eggs on a medium heat, and tip the pan just enough to let the loose egg

3. Run underneath after about one minute on the burner. Add the greens, herbs, and the seasonings to the top side as it is still soft.

4. **TIP**: You do not even have to flip it, as you can just cook the egg slowly egg as is well (being careful as not to burn).

5. **TIP**: Another option is to put it into an oven to broil for 3-5 minutes (checking to make sure it is only until it is golden but burned).

# FRAGANT ASIAN HOTPOT

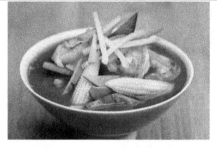

**Prep Time:** 10 mins **Cook Time:** 35 mins **Total Time:** 45 mins

## SERVING:6

### *INGREDIENTS*

- 1 tsp tomato purée
- 1-star anise, squashed (or 1/4 tsp ground anise)
- Little modest bunch (0.5 oz.) parsley, follows finely hacked
- Small, modest bunch (0.5 oz.) coriander, follows finely hacked
- Juice of 1/2 lime
- 500ml chicken stock, new or made with 1 shape
- 1/2 carrot, stripped and cut into matchsticks
- 2 oz. broccoli, cut into little florets
- 2 oz. beansprouts
- 3.5 oz. crude tiger prawns
- 3.5 oz. firm tofu, cleaved
- 2 oz. rice noodles, cooked by bundle guidelines

- 2 oz. cooked water chestnuts, depleted
- 1 oz. sushi ginger, cleaved
- 1 tbsp excellent quality miso glue

## ***INSTRUCTIONS***

1. Spot the tomato purée, star anise, parsley stalks, coriander stalks, lime juice, and chicken stock in an enormous dish and bring to a stew for 10 minutes.
2. Add the carrot, broccoli, prawns, tofu, noodles, and water chestnuts and stew tenderly until the prawns are cooked through. Eliminate from the heat and mix in the sushi ginger and miso glue.
3. Serve sprinkled with the parsley and coriander leaves.